CHATTER: Small Talk, Charisma, and
How to Talk to Anyone
(The Communication Skills & People
Skills for Success)

By Patrick King

So... how about that weather we're having today?

My friend Henry recently told me the story about how he got his current job, as he attributes it all to his small talk skills. He saw a job posting that asked for 5 years of relevant experience where he only had 3, as well as proficiency in a few hard skills in which his skill level could best be described as "I've *heard* of those..." Needless to say, he was competing against candidates that were far more qualified that he was. Even though he obtained an interview, he knew it was still a long shot.

On the day of the interview, Henry planned to arrive at the interview location 20 minutes early to go over some last minute notes he had written out. He stopped for a quick espresso from a nearby Starbucks. He got into line behind a middle-aged man in a black suit and was reading his notes to himself over and over.

The middle-aged man turned around and caught a glimpse of Henry's notes, which happened to have the company name doodled across the top of the page. He introduced himself and asked Henry why he had that name scrawled across his notes, and Henry told him that he had an interview with them shortly. The man asked why he would ever want to work there, and Henry told him honestly that he had heard great things, ranging from the management to the potential for growth and learning. He went on to say that he thought he was a perfect fit for the job, and noted a couple of problems the company currently had that he had solutions for. The man considered his answer, and switched topics, eventually learning about his fiercely proud father, agrarian upbringing, and biggest accomplishments in life thus far.

Possibly because he was nervous, because he simply wasn't concerned with what a random man at Starbucks thought of him, or just enjoyed connecting with strangers, Henry gave him long, honest answers that were thoughtful, introspective, and smart. Finally, he told him that he really cared and wanted the job, and needed to concentrate, so bid the man adieu and went in for his interview with only 2 minutes to spare.

Next week, Henry got a phone call that offered him the job, and asked to put him on hold momentarily. After waiting a few minutes, a familiar voice got on the phone and asked how his fiercely proud father would take the news of landing the job. Guess who was on the phone, who had pulled for Henry even though there were much better qualified candidates? You guessed – the man in the black suit from Starbucks, who happened to be one of the vice presidents of the company.

My name is Patrick King, and I'm a dating and image coach. My career and lifestyle has always followed the connections I was able to leverage, and you could even say that my career is heavily dependent on my charisma quotient and my ability to instantly connect with people. As you might have guessed, an immense part of this stems my capacity for that dreaded phrase we all hate: small talk.

Henry was able to succeed because he was able to connect with someone in a way that made his inferior qualifications irrelevant. Most people can learn the necessary technical skills, but we're not going to like everyone or deem them a good fit.

What about for those of us in less people-centric occupations and lifestyles... wait, those simply don't exist!

It doesn't matter if you're a computer engineer that stares at a laptop screen for 10 hours a day. You still interact with people in your social life, go out with friends, and mingle at cocktail parties.

You don't have a social life? You still wait in line while waiting for the cash register.

You do all your grocery shopping online? You still need to interview for a job and talk with co-workers to support your online shopping addiction.

So as you can see, the skill of **chatter** – being able to talk to people and connect with them – is paramount to all of us in all walks of our lives. Indulging our social sensibilities is as necessary and essential as eating and sleeping. If you can learn to make a great impression and deep connections with people that you come into contact with in your daily life, there are immeasurable benefits, such as:

1. Better interviews for getting the job you want
2. Leapfrogging better candidates for jobs because people like you more
3. Befriending people from all walks of life
4. Rising above office politics

5. An improved love life
6. Becoming the life of any party
7. Diffusing difficult situations for yourself or between others
8. Closer friendships and more intimate relationships
9. Being sought out by others
10. Improved service and occasional freebies from your waiter, deliveryman, valet... CPA, lawyer, bank...

Consider this a long-winded way of stating a universal truth: people will run through walls for people they like. If you are on someone's good side, you can punch their dog and still be loved. People are thrust forward in life by who they know... and who *likes* them!

Through years of studying human interaction and taking dozens of clients through date and image coaching, I've developed 20 Chatter Principles that will teach you exactly how to be that person in any situation. Small talk will come as natural to you as breathing. You'll learn the secrets to building a charismatic and magnetic presence. Your people skills, interpersonal and emotional intelligence will be undeniable. You will foster instant connections with people you don't know.

This isn't a book of 50 pithy conversation topics, nor are there generic tips you can find in any blog article. Chatter requires a very finely-tuned sense of empathy, conversational techniques, and cultivating a presence – it's not about just going down a checklist of topics. It also requires reading between the lines of what people say, examining body language, and noting patterns of human interaction to different types of stimuli. At some level, it's really a science, and I've laid it out as such.

Each Principle embodies a separate essential part of the interaction – either by the mindset, specific techniques, or logistical issues like entry and exit into a conversation. Taken together, these are elements that will create a powerful impression on anyone.

Principle 1: Bulletproof Your Nonverbal First Impression.

You hear it all the time. Impressions, whether fair or not, are made within 30 seconds of meeting someone.

Let's chew on that for a second. An impression of you, based on nothing but quickly observing your mannerisms, body language, appearance, and tone of speaking, influences the vast majority of your relationship with someone. Sometimes even before you say a single word! At the very least, it will certainly drive the rest of that first meeting, as your conversation partner will only pay attention to cues and signs that confirm that impression, and ignore the rest.

Simultaneously, your first impression on someone new will instantly reduce you to one simple adjective. It can be positive, negative, or worst of all, you can simply be "nice" – an afterthought with no impression. As I mentioned, it may not be fair, but it's a realistic assessment of what happens in the real world.

So how do we bulletproof our first impression, and ensure that the adjective we're reduced to is positive and glowing? First let's look at exactly what we're bulletproofing.

There are two separate components of a first impression, each as important as the other. There is a non-verbal component in which your first impression depends on your overall appearance and body language. And, as you might have guessed already, there is also a verbal component of your first impression which is governed by the way you speak, and the first 10 words out of your mouth. I'll expand on each in turn.

The handshake.

Almost without fail, the first thing you do when meeting someone new is shake their hand. It sounds simple, but there are so many ways it can go wrong. I can't tell you how many floppy fish handshakes I've received in the past year, and what that made me think of the giver. On the other side, I've also received handshakes that were way too aggressive that tried to crush my hand and insecurely assert a kind of dominance over me. Therefore, there are a few simple steps you need to follow for giving a proper handshake.

1. Offer your hand first. If there's any ambiguity about whether or not you are in handshake territory, you've just broken it and shown a willingness to connect and touch. Own and control the interaction. Being the first to offer a friendly gesture has a way of breaking down people's walls.
2. Take a step in towards them with your right leg (assuming you are right-handed) and lean in when you offer your hand. Meet them at least 50% of the way. Making them come to you is often an attempt at asserting

dominance – mostly between two males. This is, of course, stupid.

3. Find and maintain eye contact as soon as your hand goes out. Hold a smile throughout.

4. Shake their hand. Keep your hand perfectly perpendicular to the floor, and don't tilt one way or the other. Keep a stiff wrist. The tricky part is always how much pressure to use, so here's my pressure trick. Grab 2 books, short novels or otherwise and hold them in your right hand, with your arm slack at your side. The pressure that you're using to keep the books in your grip – increase that a tiny bit, and that's your handshake pressure!

5. Follow and accentuate the natural motion of a handshake – that is, slight upswing, downswing, upswing. Only one each, and then disengage and step back.

<u>Your appearance.</u>

If the world we live in is one thing, it's shallow. Just like the entire concept of a first impression, it may not be fair, but it is realistic. So what does this mean for you?

Your wardrobe must be on point. This is largely contextual, but you should always dress to the occasion, and dress to impress. You have a fancy cocktail party to go to? Women: don't go in skinny jeans and a cardigan, and men: don't go in cargo pants and a baggy collared shirt. Consider whether clothes even fit you well. The same goes for your grooming and hair. Your overall appearance is a topic for another book, but just being aware that snap judgments can and will be made can be a powerful realization in bulletproofing your first impression.

<u>Your body language</u>.

You started with your smile when you gave that handshake. Now what else about the way you carry yourself will reflect strongly and positively on anyone that even looks at you? Let's consider the following cheat sheet with steps you can implement in the next 5 minutes.

1. How's your posture? Imagine that there is a rope attached to your solar plexus, and pulling directly up. This causes your head to tilt back and your chest to push out, and is a shortcut to confident and powerful posture.

2. Have an open, approachable stance. This means that you don't cross your arms, move back from the person you are talking to, or turn away from the person you are talking to. Keep your hands out of your pockets.

3. Be aware of your nervous ticks, and either eliminate them or replace them with something more subtle. Nervous ticks exist because they are an outlet for the energy created by anxiety, whether good or bad, so I find that having a sneaky outlet for that energy, such as holding a pen, can work wonders for your appearance.

4. I already mentioned eye contact, and will do so multiple times throughout this book, but look people in the eye when you talk to them, and don't scan the room behind them while looking for someone else to talk to.

Finally, engage your eyebrows, because that's what can often make or break a facial expression.

5. Slow your movements down. Remember how fast you unintentionally talked the last time you made a speech? That's the same thing that will happen to your body language when faced with a new situation. So make your movements intentional, and attempt to move at only 75% of your normal speed, because that will probably cause it to be just about your normal speed in real life.

<u>What your conversation partner will think</u>: This person had their stuff together! I haven't even spoken to them yet, but they *look* like the type of person I want to get to know!

Principle 2: Bulletproof Your Verbal First Impression.

Luckily, your verbal first impression indicators are going to be a bit easier to bulletproof than your non-verbal indicators. You can't always control the tone and sound of your voice, but you can absolutely control *what* you say and *how* you say it.

The verbal first impression governs the first 10-20 words out of your mouth. That means your verbal first impression is almost entirely dependent on your elevator pitch. An elevator pitch is a summary about yourself and your defining characteristics tied up in a charming and funny wrapper. It is short enough to be said within the length of a normal elevator ride, in other words around 10-20 seconds, because any longer and people will get bored. The point is to keep it short, snappy, and

100% on point with zero irrelevant chatter.

To bulletproof your verbal first impression, you've got to anticipate the first 2 questions or topics of conversation that will arise with someone new, craft an elevator pitch relating to it, and rehearse it until you can say it confidently to anyone.

It turns out anticipating opening questions and topics to prepare elevator pitches for is fairly easy, so I've provided a list for you to prepare for:

1. "Tell me about yourself."

"Hey, I'm Jim. I went to school in Chicago, and arrived in Los Angeles about 2 years ago. I'm currently a photographer and office manager for a small business near Hollywood, and I seriously live to surf and play beach volleyball."

2. "What did you do last weekend?"
3. "Where do you work/what do you do?"
4. "What do you have planned for this weekend?"
5. "Do you live around here?"
6. "How do you know the person who introduced us?"
7. "Where are you from?"
8. "Where did you go to school?"

Focus on using specific details that people can relate to, as well as the commonality that you share with the person at the moment (such as the location, and the host of the party).

As with the Principle before, practice slowing down your speech to about 75% of your normal speed… because that will end up sounding normal when you're nervous or otherwise uneasy.

<u>What your conversation partner will think</u>: This person was so well put-together and confident on who they are! I'm so impressed that they lead such an interesting life… and a little jealous!

Principle 3: WWJD? What Would Jay Do?

Mastering chatter, above all else, is a matter of having the correct mindset and approach towards the people you meet. You can be the smoothest, funniest person in the room, but if you aren't *interested and curious* about your conversation partner, there simply won't be a connection.

I've found, through years of clients, that the absolute best mindset to emulate is talk show host Jay Leno's. What would Jay do? Let's think about the traits he embodies in a conversation with a guest on his show.

Visualize his studio. He's got a big open space, and he is seated at a desk. His guest is seated at a chair adjacent to the desk, and it's literally like they exist in a world of their own. When Jay has a guest on his show, that guest is the center of his world for the next 10 minutes. They are the most interesting person he has ever come across, everything they say is spellbinding, he is insatiably curious about their stories, and he reacts to anything they say with an uproarious laugh and otherwise exaggerated reaction that they were seeking. He is charmingly positive, and can always find a humorous spin on a negative aspect of a story.

His sole purpose is to make his guest comfortable on the show, talk about themselves, and ultimately make them feel good and look good. In turn, this makes them share revealing things they might not otherwise, and create a connection and chemistry with him that is so important for a talk show. The viewers at home can tell in an instant if either party is mailing it in or faking it, so his job literally depends on his ability to connect on a deeper level.

Even with grumpy or more quiet guests, he is able to elevate their energy levels and attitudes simply by being intensely interested in them (at an energy level slightly above theirs), and encouraging them by giving them the great reactions that they seek. Of course, in your life, this equates to those people you come across that are like pulling teeth to talk to. A little bit of friendly encouragement and affirmation can make even the meekest clam open up! So acting this way is beneficial for both parties. Imagine the relief you can create at dreaded networking events. People like those who like them, so when you react the way they want, it encourages them to be more outgoing and open with you.

My message here is simple. Making a decision to be genuinely curious and interested in your conversation partner is one of the keys to allowing them to feel comfortable enough to connect to you beyond a superficial level. So whether you have to fake it 'til you make it, Jay Leno is who your mindset and attitude should feel like. Everyone has something to teach you, fascinate you with, and amaze you with. Be committed to truly learning about the people you speak with, and wonder what they truly are like.

Finally, you know what Jay doesn't do while he has a guest on? Fiddle with his phone.

Dale Carnegie said it best – "You can make more friends in two months by becoming truly interested in other people than you can in two years by trying to get other people interested in you."

<u>What your conversation partner will think</u>: This was an amazing conversation! I got to show off a little bit and talk about who I really am – and they totally understood me!

Principle 4: Your Life is a Series of (Mini) Stories.

No, seriously. We don't think of our lives as being very interesting on a day to day basis, but the truth is that we do quite a bit more than we realize. This proposition, combined with the fact that nothing stops a conversation cold quite like a one word answer, means that you should strive to make your life a series of mini stories. This is also a chance to control the kind of image you want to project to your conversation partner, by finding the right experiences from your life to use.

Stories are an inside view to your personality, emotions, passions. Learning those about you is the first step in allowing anyone to relate and feel connected to you, so it's imperative that you learn how to take a close-ended question and expand it to your advantage. It will also encourage them to reciprocate, and suddenly trading war stories from college parties is on the table. Your goal should be to hear "Wait until you hear what happened to me!" from your conversation partner at least once.

This is going to require you to take a mental survey of the aspects of yourself that you want to highlight, then and making sure that it's something that is objectively interesting. To make that distinction clear, it's the difference between being proud of your video game prowess and being proud of your new artwork.

"So what do you do?"
"I'm a marketing executive. It's pretty cool!"
"Oh, nice."

Let's try again.

"So what do you do?"
"I'm a marketing executive. I deal mostly with clients… just last week we

had a crazy client that threatened to send his bodyguards to our office! I definitely wish I dealt more with the creative side." "Oh, my God! Did he actually send them?"

See how the second example contains so much more substance for them to connect with, to avoid interview mode, and make conversation flow more smoothly? The next natural step in the conversation above is to organically talk about the crazy client and other funny aspects of work, instead of awkwardly playing "Now how about you?"

I implore you to cue up similar mini stories (~3 sentences) for some of the most common conversation topics that will arise, such as:

1. Your occupation (if you have a job that is unusual or nebulous, make sure that you have a layman's description of your job that people can relate to)
2. Your week
3. Your upcoming weekend

4. Your hometown
5. Your hobbies
6. Your favorite music
7. Your passions
8. Your education
9. Your apartment/house
10. Your mutual friends
11. Your dating history
12. Your experience with the venue you're at
13. The weather
14. Your family
15. Your pet

As you can see from my example, don't just answer the question directly. Make it a mini story that can stand by itself. Again, check if they portray you to be what you want as your image. Just don't get too personal, negative, or controversial, and don't dominate the conversation.

<u>What your conversation partner will think</u>: There isn't a boring bone in this person's body! I'm going to make it a goal to become friends with them so I can be included in the next crazy story.

Principle 5: Thorough, Exhaustive, and Specific Details.

Let's examine the following scenario where you've just met Glen.

"Hi Glen, nice to meet you. What do you do?"
"Engineering stuff."
"Interesting." (with faked enthusiasm)

This is exactly the moment where you realize that talking to Glen is going to be a chore. How could Glen have answered better? Maybe something specific and detailed, such as:

"Oh, I'm a software engineer and I'm currently working on a project to find out how to schedule a day of movie-hopping within a theater."
"Interesting!" (with real enthusiasm)

Just as a one word answer is the death knell for any conversation, a reply or question devoid of any detail castrates a conversation. You are to never use the phrases "I don't know," "Nothing much," or "Just hangin' out" again! The way to avoid being a Glen (sorry if your name is Glen) is simply to insert personal details into a conversation.

The typical trend in a surface conversation is to just ask out of courtesy about people, so once you lead with a specific detail that begs to be asked about, the trend is bucked and the conversation immediately takes a life of its own. In the same vein, you should be graphic, and use extremely descriptive and colorful language.

Regarding perception, think beyond the conversation. If someone asks you about Glen, you wouldn't have much to say about him at all besides the fact that he was nice. But if you drop personal details that are interesting and funny, your conversation partner will know and remember you through them. Would you rather be Jim the nice guy, or Jim the guy who just had a deer attack him? This provides a few benefits when you examine the structure of a conversation:

1. It creates a direction for the conversation to follow.
2. It encourages asking about the detail, and straying from having the same conversation as you do with anyone else.
3. It creates a potential commonality for your conversation partner to bond over. You can also ensure that the details you divulge are relatable.
4. It makes the conversation easier to continue for your conversation partner. Conversations are a give and take, and you want to make it as easy on your partner as possible.
5. Finally and most importantly, it creates a personal connection and encourages your conversation partner to reciprocate. People like people who are similar to them, and details open the avenue to that discovery.

As you can see, a simple detail can have a huge impact on how well an interaction goes, and takes almost no effort on your part. This Principle is similar to the previous Principle of using mini stories whenever possible, but is a way to construct the mini stories themselves.

If you find that you struggle to provide any sort of details to someone who is inquiring, then it might be time to take a look at yourself objectively and determine whether that is something that needs to change.

<u>What your conversation partner will think</u>: I feel like I really know some intimate details about her life, and that really allowed me to divulge some of my own.

Principle 6: Icebreak with Superficial Commonalities…

Next time you're at a party, make a mental checklist of the questions you are asked by your new acquaintances. Chances are that they are shallow, cursory questions that only serve to discover what *superficial commonalities* you both share. They jump from topic to topic, and don't take into account any details. If you meet more than 3 people in a single night, you'll be struck with the oddest sense of déjà vu that you've had this exact conversation before…

For example:

"Hey Juan, great to meet you. Where did you go to school?"

"You too, Jimbo! I went to Ohio State University."

"Oh cool! What do you do now?"

You might as well walk around with a nametag on your shoulder with your vital statistics, education, occupation, blood type, and hometown all listed. Of course, none of us are innocent in this either. When Juan said that he went to Ohio State University, we all had a slight cringe inside because we hoped that he went to the same college that we did, or that our brother did, or that their our friend Wendy did.

Hunting for superficial commonalities is a great way to begin conversations on a daily basis, and they are common icebreakers for a reason. None of us can expect to be charming, witty, and engaged 100% of the time, so more often than not, we rely on the superficial hunt.

But there is an *optimal* way to do so that can lead to some interesting revelations and avoid ticking the boxes on your nametag.

First, it is important to realize that your gender can play a huge part in which superficial commonalities you should target aside from the norm. At this point, I feel like I should offer a disclaimer in which I state that I cannot reduce entire genders to 4-5 interests, nor generalize my experiences to everyone. I should also state that your experiences may tell you differently, and that you should go with your gut if that's the case. Finally, I'm not a sexist.

That said, there are specific topics I've found that are simply the easiest icebreakers to lead with, depending on who you are and who you are talking to. They are topics that there is mutual interest in, and that they will almost certainly feel comfortable talking about. If need be, fall back on these topics as defaults.

For a man talking to a man, the bailiwick topics are: women, sports, work/business, working out, food, and vehicles. Now you see why I added a disclaimer above. For a woman talking to a woman, the bailiwick topics are: physical appearance (your/her clothing, hair, etc.), recent events they have attended, food, and other women. Finally, when talking to the opposite sex, the bailiwick topics are: working out, events they have attended, mutual friends.

Second, not all icebreakers are created equal. Try to stray away from the typical personality traits such as hobbies, interests, and occupation for two reasons. First, you'll inevitably learn those facts about the person organically sooner or later, and don't have to ask them directly. Second, people are so used to answering them that they give canned answers because they are bored and unstimulated.

A really great icebreaker on superficial commonalities is related to the mutual shared reality at hand, and how you address them with your conversation partner. (A technique pioneered by Carol Fleming, renowned author)

1. Discover what you two share at the moment. It could be a location, mutual friend, interest, looking at the

same piece of art, shoes, tapping your foot to the background music, you name it. If you don't see a shared reality with someone, you're not looking hard enough.

2. Reveal something about yourself related to that shared reality. Focus on yourself, and whatever relation or context you have with it.

3. Prompt your conversation partner with the reveal. Use the personal information from step 2 to make a statement or question prompt your partner to reply, gauge their reaction, share their own relation, and get them involved.

It's as simple as seeing someone tapping their foot to the music, and saying "I love this band, they just came through Chicago last week and I can't believe I missed them!"

<u>What your conversation partner will think</u>: I can't believe I found someone at this party that grew up in the same hometown as me! And that has the same 2 favorite bands! We'll hang out for sure.

Principle 7: But Core Commonalities Foster True Relationships.

As I previously discussed, superficial commonalities are a great way to jumpstart a conversation. They are not, however, ideal for building deep connections and relationships that will get you where you want to go. It can be done, but there are simply much better ways to do it. Instead of focusing on superficial commonalities, focusing on core commonalities takes you on a shortcut to someone's inner circle.

What exactly is a core commonality, versus a superficial one?

<u>A core commonality is a trait, emotion, feeling, formative experience... fear, insecurity, vulnerability, or aspiration you have in common with someone else</u>.

Notice that these are things that are deeply important to people, and often a defining characteristic. It creates a far more powerful connection than simply having gone to the same college, because it allows a few assumptions about the other person, whether fairly or unfairly.

The first assumption is that they are on your level status-wise, however you define the word. This is a powerful psychological component in being interested and curious in what someone has to say. If you feel that someone is the same status as you, or even slightly higher, you're simply going to want to make a good impression on them and connect more. This bodes well for any conversation.

The second assumption is that you are both privy to exclusive knowledge and experiences. The two of you inhabit a world that no one else knows about, so a strong bond is immediately created on the basis of sharing that specialized knowledge or experience. And just as with the first assumption, there is a psychological effect that is created that makes opening up and connecting all the easier.

The third and final assumption when a core commonality is discovered is that besides status, you are simply similar to them as a whole. People like people like themselves, it's a simple fact. People will also seek out others like themselves, be more likely to help others like themselves, and seek to integrate them into their friend circles.

So as you can see, introducing a core commonality has been the basis for many a lasting friendship. Now the natural question is how to get to them. This is best seen through example.

Here's how a conversation focused on superficial commonalities sounds like, which, as we discussed, is a good starting point for many contexts:

"Oh wow, you were born in New York too?" "Yeah!"

"What part?" "Brooklyn, what about you?"
"Buffalo." "Oh, awesome. I have an uncle that lives there."
"Nice. Did you go to school there too?"

See how quickly that potential gold mine of a topic of New York is closed shut? Now here's a conversation that is more focused on core commonalities:

"Oh wow, you were born in New York too?" "Yeah, Brooklyn born and raised!" "Awesome, I've always wanted to spend more time there. Did you go to a PS (public high school) there?" "Yeah, public school all the way! You too?" "Definitely, it shaped me! I liked growing up with a little bit of edge." "Yeah, I completely agree. One time when I was a kid…"

Within 3 sentences, they've connected on a deep level about their childhoods, and dipped into formative experiences that relatively few people can share and relate to. They ask probing questions, reveal personal experiences, and really emphasize an obscure yet important commonality. The focus also tends to be on one person initially, without a "What about you?" back and forth – those details will inevitably surface later in the conversation. Don't jump from one topic to the next. Finally, keeping previous Principles in mind, the way each question is answered provides detail and stories.

<u>What your conversation partner will think</u>: This guy is like my brother! Did I get his phone number? Because I definitely need to hang out with him again and introduce him to my friends.

Principle 8: Know and Play in Your Wheelhouse.

I watch Jeopardy!, a trivia show, fairly often. There's no way to watch it except with amazement at the seemingly unlimited knowledge that the contestants possess. Imagine how easy it would be to talk to any of them, because of the sheer knowledge they possess and the range of topics they would be able to connect with you on.

Therein lies a simple truth that we can take advantage of: the more you know about a topic, the easier it is to talk to someone about it, whether by explaining, teaching, discussing, or debating. For us mere mortals, we can dabble in some topics, but we all have main topics and strengths where our knowledge lies – our wheelhouse topics. Logically, there is only one conclusion we can draw from this. Know what your wheelhouse topics are, and play to them!

First, put yourself under a microscope and honestly think about topics and realms of knowledge that you feel comfortable talking to in any situation. It might be as short a list as "makeup, shopping, French food, and soccer" and that's fine. This may seem limiting, but the next step will show how to get the most out of your wheelhouse topics, expand them, and ultimately become comfortable talking about anything.

Second, let's visualize both a Russian babushka doll and a model of an atom. The Russian doll is composed of layers of dolls that fit inside each other. The smallest doll is your most specific wheelhouse topic that you can expound on for hours. Each subsequent, larger doll is a slightly more general category than the one inside it.

By contrast, the atom model has a central nucleus, with orbiting protons, electrons and neutrons. Your main wheelhouse topic is the nucleus, and the surrounding particles are all related, but not necessarily more general categories. Let's illustrate the two approaches with a kind of flowchart.

The Russian doll method: The Beatles >> 60's music >> classic pop music >> rock bands >> music.

The atom method: soccer >> competition >> working out >> sports >> running.

So while the goal here has been to visualize how you can pivot a conversation to one of your wheelhouse topics, this exercise exponentially increases the ways you can do it within a conversation. If we take the example from above, with four topics consisting of "makeup, shopping, French food, and soccer," we see how we can easily expand it to over 20 topics that we feel comfortable talking about and breaking ice with.

It's worth mentioning that this is a relatively beginner technique that's ideal for those that have trouble connecting and conversing on topics outside of their comfort zones. It's meant to allow you to gradually branch out as you discover just how easy it is to relate to things not immediately in your wheelhouse, even as the connections grow more and more tenuous. A simple "That reminds me…" or "Last time I played soccer…" or "What about…" is all it takes to get back to a wheelhouse topic.

It's also worth mentioning that doing this constantly will transform you into the most self-absorbed person at the party, as opposed as someone who simply plays to their strengths. It will take practice to learn when you need to do this, when you should resist the urge, and when the natural flow of the conversation opens itself up to it.

Finally, imagine the comfort and security you might feel wash over you as a bailiwick topic comes up. Now turn the tables and imagine the comfort and security that you can make others feel, especially quieter and more reserved people, by directing the conversation to topics that are in *their* wheelhouse. Strive to give value as a conversation partner!

<u>What your conversation partner will think</u>: Wow, she could talk about any topic that came up. She's a seriously smart and cultured person.

Principle 9: Reactions are Worth 1,000 Words.

Conversation-wise, there's no greater pleasure than having someone know exactly the point that you're trying to convey. Everyone loves to be agreed with. This person understands exactly how it feels to lose 100 lbs in 6 months too?! It imparts the feeling that you're really being listened to, and you may have even found a kindred spirit. Of course, true kindred spirits are few and far between, and so are people that actually can relate to the obscure experience you're talking about. So how do you get someone to really feel like you are listening to them and can relate to the words coming out of their mouths?

Great, big, juicy reactions.

The meaning of a reaction in the conversation context isn't immediately apparent to most people, and most people don't even realize that they're doing it at all. But when the reactions stop, you'll notice how much less a conversation flows, and how awkward and robotic the other person suddenly becomes. Great reactions are like the soundtrack to any movie – they accentuate the scene at hand, drive the plot along, and make the viewer truly understand the context and background of the story. Without the soundtrack, the movie suddenly becomes curiously disjointed and generally flat.

So then, what exactly is a conversation reaction? There are verbal and non-verbal reactions, both of which are vital to any reaction.

Verbal reactions can be as simple as saying "Oh, really," "Sure…" "Oh yeah?" "Dang!" "Whoa…" "No kidding?" "Go on…" "No way!" or gasping in disbelief. Arguably the most important reaction is laughter, especially when the speaker is expecting it or laughing themselves. They are acknowledgments or leading questions that let the speaker know that you have heard them, are interested in them continuing, and want to hear more.

They also amplify the emotions that the speaker is trying to convey, simply by agreeing and prodding them to continue. This has the effect of exciting the speaker and raising the overall energy and emotional level of the conversation, which is vital for a connection to form. If you're having trouble with this, practice by having reactions and your inner monologue out loud that you'd normally have only mentally.

The key to both verbal and non-verbal reactions is simply to learn to know which reactions your conversation partner is seeking, and give it to them in a subtle way. Much of it is matching their reactions and tone.

Let's look at some non-verbal reactions to see some clear illustrations.

1. When your conversation partner talks about something disapprovingly, shake your head and grimace.
2. When your conversation partner asks a rhetorical question, smile and shake your head to show that you understand.
3. When your conversation partner is explaining something, tilt your head and squint your eyes to make a thinking and processing face.
4. When your conversation partner talks about something that made them mad, facepalm and shake your head.
5. When your conversation partner says something they aren't sure about, tilt your head to the side and squint your eyes questioningly.
6. When you conversation partner poses a question that you identify with, nod your head emphatically and throw your head back with a grin.
7. When your conversation partner talks about something that surprised them, pretend to pull out your hair and widen your eyes as much as possible.
8. When your conversation partner is explaining something obtuse to you,

show concentration by furrowing your brows and tilting your head.

Obviously, these will vary from person to person. But the common thread, as you can see, is to try to read the emotion your partner is trying to evoke, and display it to them.

<u>What your conversation partner will think</u>: I really felt like that guy understood what I was trying to convey, even though no one else really does.

Principle 10: Cold Reads Accelerate Any
Conversation.

"You're a Virgo, aren't you?"

"I bet you can't sit still during movies."

"You seem like the type of person that
wrestled in high school."

"So when's the last time you ran a
marathon?"

Enter the cold read. A cold read is a
statement or question that makes a bold
assumption about your conversation
partner based on something they have
said previously in the same conversation.
It can follow logically from their
previous statement, or it can just be a
non-sequitur that you impose on them. It
doesn't really matter which way you
decide to go – if you're correct about the
assumption you make, then you're

suddenly as perceptive as Sherlock Holmes and extremely insightful.

If you're wrong about the assumption, then you've opened up an entertaining line of conversation that wouldn't have existed otherwise. More often than not, you'll probably be right. Either way, the conversation inevitably takes a turn for the unique and better. Let's take a look at how this plays out to see how we can effectively utilize a cold read.

"Ugh, I can't believe that that steak was so overcooked!"

Cold read: "You're a big foodie, aren't you?"

You'll typically get 1 of 3 reactions to your cold read.

#1: "Yeah... how did you know?"

#2: "Maybe…"

#3: "Not at all! Where did you get that idea?"

As I discussed, any of these reactions will spiral the conversation into an exciting direction with distinct explanations, stances, and backstories. An opinion and assertion is created, which is conversation dynamite. Finally, using hyperbole in your assumption can lead to big laughs ("Do you wish you were Gordon Ramsay?"). It's a refreshing alternative to exchanging "what about you's".

You should be cautious however, that without a big grin and some congruent body language, using a cold read can come across as rude and invasive. Again, it's a matter of practicing reading the situation and the person, and knowing how a cold read will be taken by them.

<u>What your conversation partner will think</u>: That girl read me like a book! So smart and perceptive.

Principle 11: Listening Effectively is like Giving Out Truth Serum.

"So… how does that make you feel?"

Parroted by psychologists and comic strip artists all around the world, it turns out that there is good reason for its prevalence. This statement is representative of a communication technique called active listening, and when done correctly, can lead someone to shine a torch into their own soul. Active listening is most often used by therapists and counselors, so it's not a technique for normal, everyday conversations, and is better suited towards serious topics and serious settings. As this Principle is titled, listening effectively is like giving out truth serum.

Active listening is characterized by the following:

1. Focusing on other person.
2. Staying on a limited amount of topics.
3. Rephrasing, paraphrasing, or simply repeating what the other person said to confirm your perception and understanding and make them expand.
4. Asking the right questions to dig deeper.
5. Gradually zeroing in on the underlying issue at hand.
6. Having the other person examine their own true intents.
7. Frequent epiphanies.

When all 6 of the above are achieved, it's really quite something to see. Paraphrasing someone's words and making assumptions based on what they've said invariably makes them elaborate their position, and clarify it on a deeper level to show underlying thoughts. If you go through enough iterations and are fortunate enough to ask the right questions, you can suddenly end up at the root cause of someone's insecurities, relationship troubles, or career struggles. Let's see a short session of active listening and what it can lead to.

"I think I've finally decided that I want to practice copyright law!"
"Oh, why is that?"
"I just think it's a good mix of constitutional rights and innovation!"
"Where exactly is innovation in copyright law?"
"Well, you know there are lots of cases involving big tech companies like YouTube and Google, so that's cool."
"It sounds like you might just be interested in working with tech, rather than copyright?"
"Well, I like both, but copyright touches a lot more than just tech – like photography and writing, which are some of my favorite hobbies."
"You seem to care about the subject matter rather than copyright itself."
"I don't know, I just like the idea of copyrights... I guess it's the creativity involved."

"Sounds to me that you're just drawn to it because there are aspects of creativity, which you enjoy as hobbies."
"That's a good point…"

Epiphany reached. As you can see in this extremely abbreviated snippet, the active listener encouraged the speaker to mentally wander and think out loud by paraphrasing and asking questions that challenged what the speaker said. Then, when the opportunity was there, the active listener was able to zero in on the root of the speaker's intentions and help the speaker reach that conclusion himself.

It should be noted that the speaker did all the talking and all the work in getting to that point, and the active listener merely acted as a sounding board. Encourage them to get technical about their work or otherwise, because they will cherish the opportunity to teach someone about their field of expertise.

Key phrases to use during active listening are:

1. You seem to feel…
2. It sounds to me like...
3. What I'm hearing is…
4. So, you're…
5. So… (repeat the last few words they just said)
6. And is that because…

You can easily imagine how each of those prompts can cause someone to reflect on what they've said and clarify it even further. It will take practice to do effectively, but active listening is a shockingly powerful communication technique once mastered.

While on the subject of listening effectively, I want to impart my most powerful piece of advice to make people feel heard. After someone speaks, nod your head thoughtfully and *pause for 2 full seconds before you speak or react*. Do not simply launch into what you were going to say, and do not ignore the points that they have made. An intentional pause will give the appearance that you've really heard what they've said, and are taking extra time to absorb and address it. It makes clear that you are not simply waiting for your turn to speak, which is an extremely frustrating feeling to battle.

<u>What your conversation partner will think</u>: Oh my God, she just peered into my soul and led me to the answers I was looking for! I got incepted!

Principle 12: Skew Slightly Inappropriate.

I have a gay friend named Ben, and Ben has the gift of being able to say absolutely whatever he wants to anyone. It's irrelevant that he's gay, but it certainly helps the visualization. He doesn't quite have the gift of gab, but he can say the most inappropriate, lewd statement or question, and people typically eat it up and play along.

He might exclaim something like "Nice tits today, bitch!" to a male or male friend, and the reaction is always positive and humorous.

I'm not telling you to go about commenting on the sexual characteristics of your friends. But there's something to be said for Ben's lack of propriety and how it really opens up people and puts them at ease.

The root of the hesitancy and awkwardness of small talk is that people are afraid of saying the wrong thing and alienating their conversation partner. It's always a dance of sugarcoating because you just don't know what your conversation partner is like. This in turn causes anxiety, nervousness, and general fumbling over words. Skewing inappropriate in your conversation immediately gets that out of the way, and both parties can essentially breathe a sigh of relief and relax. It's like how you can lighten up and relax when your substitute teacher drops a swear sword casually – you just know that he's going to be a relaxed and open person. People are typically far less uptight and mature than we give them credit for, and people always skew inappropriate with their friends. So by doing so, it opens up a channel of comfort they often only reserve for friends.

Sex and bathroom humor often work out well, and so do doses of dark humor and sarcasm. Now for some examples to illustrate how to skew inappropriate in context. Of note, these must be said with congruent body language and smiles, or else you have just pulled off a John Wayne Gacy impression.

1. Sexual innuendos. "I can't believe I let that one inside." "Oh I bet you can, you dirty girl."
2. Colorful analogies and language. "Is that guy single?" "I don't know, but he's like Jim's masturbation hand – always ready for more."
3. Describing things in a funny yet crass way. "Sheila's not here, I think she's getting destroyed by that guy she met at the club."
4. The invasive question. "What's the weather outside?" "I haven't been outside yet this afternoon, but how was the weather in your pants on your date last night?"

The invasive question is by far the most widely usable technique because pushing on a specific topic will yield fruit. Skewing slightly inappropriate is also great for conversation because it pushes the envelope in terms of topics that are on the table, and can lead to some seriously intense or personal discussions. Done correctly, you won't be pegged as immature or one-tracked minded, simply open and slightly outrageous.

<u>What your conversation partner will think</u>: Whoa, she didn't just say that did she? That was hilarious.

Principle 13: Callback During Conversation Lulls.

If you've gotten to this point in the book, you've learned how to expertly steer a conversation in any direction you please while captivating your conversation partner. You know how to build rapport, exude charisma, and create instant connections. The problem is that a conversation works best with 2 skilled speakers, and most people won't be quite as adept as you. So regardless of every technique that you've learned to open people up and fascinate them, you will inevitably have to deal with conversation lulls and the occasional awkward silence. *C'est la vie*.

There are a variety of methods to deal with this, and most simply redirect attention back the conversation you were having in a natural way; hence the title of this Principle. The goal is to organically fill the silence, and keep the energy level and flow of the conversation high. Ideally, your lull-breakers will prompt your conversation partner to break the silence themselves.

1. "I keep thinking about what you were saying before…"
2. Start laughing, then say "I was just laughing at what you said earlier…"
3. Where did you say you were born, again?"
4. "Holy cow, look at that lampshade!"
5. "This is random, but last night I was on Netflix and spent so much time looking for something to watch that I just settled on Arrested Development for the 50th time."
6. "Hold on, I've got something in my eye…"

What's happening in each of these examples?

1. I stayed within the conversation and referred to something that they said

before. This puts the burden on them to elaborate more on the prior topic.

2. I stayed within the conversation and referred to something funny that your conversation partner said. This will make your partner launch into the story again.

3. I essentially made them repeat themselves and revisit a topic in greater detail.

4. I went outside of the conversation and brought an external talking point in. Easy to do, but can break the flow you previously had.

5. I stated a non-sequitur that I thought was funny and relatable. I would recommend having one prepared, with an emphasis on the relatable part. Just ask yourself what a common struggle is you have every day.

6. Your failsafe! If you really cannot think of something to interject.

What your conversation partner will think: There were never any conversation lulls or awkward silences! Talking to her was so easy and effortless.

Principle 14: You Are a Current Events Sponge.

As of the time of writing this book, the Sochi 2014 Winter Olympics are taking place. I cannot stand figure skating – my parents forced me to watch it instead of the 90's sitcoms I would always rather be watching, and I haven't recovered since.

But you know what? I forced myself to research the top competitors from each country with a particular emphasis on the American ice skaters. I looked up results from each round of the qualifiers, read reviews of the top performances, and manufactured an opinion on who I thought *really* should have won.

The point I'm making is that regardless of what your personal preferences are, keep up to date on any big current events that are sure to make their way into a conversation. Formulate an opinion and be able to defend it at least superficially. As I mentioned before with your wheelhouse topics, the more you know about a topic, the better equipped you are for any conversation – and that's our real goal, speaking to people and connecting with them, not to enjoy figure skating. This is one area where you can truly prepare beforehand, as opposed to thinking on your feet as many of the techniques in this book require.

Becoming a current events sponge is an easier process than you might imagine, and doesn't have to involve heavy research. My figure skating preparation ended up being overkill from my usual method of quickly assimilating a topic I have no clue about.

Patrick's method to becoming a current events sponge:

1. Skim the headlines of the front page of 3 major newspapers (or their websites). This is to get a sense of what's truly important, and make sure that nothing is missed. Focus on

politics, national events, social and media news, music, and sports.

2. Take note of the 5 biggest news stories.

3. Ask around in your friend group to see who is informed on the issues. We all have at least one friend like that, and we probably ignore most of their diatribes. But here they come in handy. Ask them for a quick rundown of the issues and ask their opinion on it.

4. Now that you're informed enough for any conversation on the topic, research an obscure fact about it. You want this to make someone say "Wow, really? I had no idea!" and add something new to a topic that most people know something about already. The obscure fact makes you seem ridiculously informed and on top of the issue.

5. Think about the crowd that you'll be going into. If you're going to a party full of musicians, bone up on the current chart toppers, do some listening, and research the origins of

a popular DJ. Calibrate to your audience.

Follow the 5 steps above and you will never be speechless again.

As it turns out, I discovered that there is more grace and athletic power in figure skating that I thought, so being a current events sponge might broaden your horizons as well.

<u>What your conversation partner will think</u>: Holy cow, that guy blew my mind with how much he knew about Obamacare, Especially the obscure point that it actually lowers costs for middle-sized businesses!

Principle 15: Charisma is a Choice.

What exactly is charisma?

I had the opportunity to meet Bill Clinton when he was traveling and promoting his autobiography. Granted, it was for less than a minute, but a powerful impression was made. If the word charisma had a picture next to it, it would be his portrait. Most definitions of charisma are just about presence and magnetism, which aren't inaccurate, but also do not help you visualize how to achieve it. So what is charisma? I can define it by how Bill Clinton made me feel. Insert crass yet obvious Monica Lewinsky joke.

<u>He made me feel like he cared about every single word I had to say.</u>

And he probably didn't, but that's beside the point. He made me feel that he was interested in what I had to say by his (1) body language, (2) eye contact, and (3) deep follow-up questions. He was friendly, welcoming, and his handshake verged on intimate. He made smiling eye contact with me for every moment he wasn't signing his book. He didn't scan the room for who was next, or check his watch for the time. He asked me where I was from, how I ended up here, and about my family. He made it sound like he wanted to meet my brother. He was fully engaged with me and me alone. He was genuine, grounded and showed compassion.

He made me feel lucky to be talking to him.

This sounds like something that you might not have control over, but that's a myth. You may not be able to imitate the intimidating visage of the former President of the United States of America, but you can certainly create your own presence and perception of influence where people will view you in a positive and (relatively) powerful light.

This is a concept known as social proof, where people observe how others react to you, and adjust their expectations and perceptions accordingly. For example, if Cameron Diaz and Tom Cruise stepped off the red carpet specifically to say hi to you, then everyone who has seen that will inflate their expectations and perception of you based on how Tom and Cameron treated you. Social proof is precisely why name-dropping is a thing.

Social proof is easily reproduced in our daily lives by observing how people react to others, how much they look forward to speaking to them, how they speak about them, and how many people talk about them – the more/better, the higher social proof and relative status you'll attain, and the more people will feel lucky when talking to you.

<u>He made me feel good about myself.</u>

At this point in his career, I'm pretty sure Bill Clinton is self-aware enough to realize the impact he has on people. He's been through enough sticky situations to intimately understand empathy, and use it to his advantage. So when I spoke with him, he was eminently aware that I was nervous and starstruck, and put me at ease immediately. He joked around with me and made a self-deprecating jab at his humble Arkansas roots. He was extremely warm and reacted extremely positively to everything I mentioned to him. Beyond the gravity of who I was speaking to, I came away from that brief conversation in an elevated mood, and with a wonderful impression of Slick Willie.

So what can we learn from Bill Clinton? There were no secrets to his amazing charisma, only precise execution and awareness. Every one of us can do what he did, it's simply a matter of recognizing and choosing to do it.

All anyone really gets out of a conversation is a combination of 3 things: entertainment, information, and pleasure. Charisma easily imparts all 3, and is a big step towards owning any room.

<u>What your conversation partner will think</u>: That woman was magnetic. I was mesmerized by everything she said, and she seemed really interested in me too!

Principle 16: Save Buzzkill Topics for the Internet.

I'm known to be a great deflector in conversations. If someone wants to bring up Afghanistan, Obamacare, or any of Africa's multitude of atrocities, I'll politely acknowledge the topic, then almost immediately switch to a topic that is more lighthearted and less controversial. There are many reasons I do this, but the big one is simply that odds are that the topic attempting to be shoehorned in is uninteresting to most people in a conversation, polarizing, and a festering ground for uninformed opinions.

"Hey, I just read that Obamacare is detrimental to small businesses, can you believe that?"

"Did you know that that meat you're eating was killed unethically?"

"I'm so against this war it's not even funny."

What kind of conversation can you really have on those topics… or any other buzzkill topic like religion, politics, illness, death, sex (sometimes), and finances? Especially when it is usually presented in such a pointed manner?

This Principle is dedicated to learning how to avoid buzzkill topics and diffusing the situations that can arise from them. Save those discussions and arguing for the Internet where you can do no harm, and where you can pound people with all the biased articles you can find.

It's important to realize the reason that most buzzkill topics are brought into a conversation at all. In my experience, there are two overriding reasons for someone to introduce the chaos of a buzzkill topic.

First, someone has undertaken the assumption that having knowledge of a buzzkill topic (and also a topic that they view as serious and mature) will make them appear informed and knowledgeable. When someone acts on that assumption, the reaction they are looking for isn't actually to have an open discourse. They are simply seeking validation, and want confirmation of their world knowledge prowess.

The second reason that most people bring up buzzkill topics is that they want to push their own agenda. Of course, this usually leaves zero room for meaningful discourse, and is often inflammatory and offensive. They just want their opinion to be heard, to convince people, and for people to agree with them.

As you can see, buzzkill topics aren't introduced to further the conversation. Seldom are deep connections made over buzzkill topics, and even more seldom will you change someone's mind at a cocktail party. As a result, they can be the death of many a conversation, and even friendship.

What does this mean for you, the charismatic small talk expert who wants conversations to flow as smooth as possible? The best way to both avoid and diffuse buzzkill topics is to appeal to their underlying vanities.

Now that we know the likely motivation of the introducer of the buzzkill topic, acknowledge and affirm it quickly, then move on! This might consist of pandering to their ego, agreeing with them, or just giving them an amazed look accompanied by a "Whoa, really?" Here's a few ways to do it.

"Hey, I just read that Obamacare is detrimental to small businesses, can you believe that?"
"Whoa, really? That's really insightful because everyone says the opposite! You're so well-informed. Wait, let me tell you about what I just read…"

"Did you know that that meat you're eating was killed unethically?"

"Dang, you know so much about so many random things. Mr. Jeopardy here. Oh, what'd you do this weekend?"

"I'm so against this war it's not even funny."

"Yeah, I know what you mean. It's crazy! Hold on… didn't you just hike Mount Verge last week?"

See how the responses are acknowledged, vanities are appealed to, then a new topic is introduced almost as a random afterthought? Occasionally you will run into someone that refuses to take the hint and keep reverting back to their buzzkill topic – in those instances, you can feel free to simply say that you don't know much about the topic and revert back to *your* topic.

The only time I would recommend staying on a buzzkill topic for longer than the time it takes you to dismiss it is if you have a truly great, positive and preferably hilarious story about it.

You just don't want to ever be in a conversation where no one is smiling, and where people are only waiting for their turn to talk.

<u>What your conversation partner will think</u>: (nothing or smug satisfaction, they will probably be oblivious)

Principle 17: Outrageous Introductions Eliminate Awkwardness.

For those of us that ride public transportation on a regular basis, you know that it can often be a laugh riot. The woman asking people where her pet hamster is fairly par for the course, along with the man that dances to Michael Jackson as if no one is watching.

Now here's something you might not have realized about Mexican Michael Jackson over there: it is shockingly easy to strike up a conversation about him with anyone that sees him. Even if it's just a shared snicker, knowing glance, or stifled grin, Miguel Jackson has massive potential to be conversation gold because he makes people react, and people innately want to react in a social manner. Of course, it can also just be a funny excuse to talk.

Put another way, imagine you have a tyrannical boss that belongs in the comic strip *Dilbert*. As soon as he finishes a particularly loud tirade, the natural reaction will be to look at your co-workers in amazement and just laugh, even if you had just met them. Having something outrageous in your sphere makes people want to confirm with others that it's really happening that validate that their feelings are appropriate, which is a purely social reaction. It's a bonding moment.

Which brings me to this Principle. When you introduce others, you should create an outrageous factor that thrusts people together. You must become the Miguel Jackson in the absence of other outrageous sights. When the focus of the conversation is on anything but the other person, even momentarily, it drastically decreases the amount of pressure to constantly talk and makes it far more comfortable and natural.

So how do you channel Miguel?

1. "Candy, have you met Ben? He bikes to work in tiny spandex every day."

I introduced them with a funny fact about one of the parties, which he will feel compelled to defend and justify and tell a story about, while she pokes fun at him.

2. "Josh, this is John. Last time I hung out with John, we ended up in the same bed together."

I pointed out a funny commonality the parties share. He will launch into the story about ending up together, and she will laugh her head off at it.

3. "Angie, this is Kenneth. You both have unfortunately seen how much body hair I have."

I made myself the butt of the joke to be laughed at. They will probably gang up on me and share stories about how bad my hair is, and the last time they both saw it.

4. "Carol, this is Charles. Carol, remember when you tore that guy's shirt off at the bar?"

I introduced a funny story about one of the parties, which she will adamantly and proudly justify while he cracks up.

5. "Steph, this is Andrew. I'm pretty sure you two have the most delicate stomachs ever."

I focused on a humorous commonality the two of them share, which will result in them comparing notes and experiences about it, no matter how gross.

6. "Nick, this is Audrey. Yes… THE Audrey." (and then you turn around and leave immediately)

I created an outrageous situation that will make Nick root around for what I meant by "THE Audrey," and Audrey listing daring things she has done. My leaving just makes it more outrageous and funny.

The point is to make them laugh to disarm them. 99% of the time when you use any of the introduction techniques in this book, there will be a related story that will kickstart their conversation. If I could sum this chapter up in one sentence, it would be this: shift the focus away from their meeting.

A bit better than swapping occupations, hometowns, and colleges, isn't it?

<u>What your conversation partner will think</u>: Oh my God, what a hilariously embarrassing way to be introduced! At least it eliminated awkward silences!

Principle 18: Don't be a Conversation Hunter or Deer.

There are few feelings more painful than being trapped like a deer by someone who is hunting for conversation partners. You're barely acknowledging them, you're scanning the room for some sort of relief, and yet they prattle on about which type of bear is best.

And yet, an even more painful feeling is if you suddenly realize that you are that person described – the conversation hunter herself!

This Principle focuses on both how to avoid (1) being the conversation deer and (2) being the conversation hunter.

Avoiding being a conversation deer and preserving your freedom to roam free between all types of conversations is easier than you might think. At our core, we all instinctually know that it can be insulting to abruptly leave or end a conversation. But leaving the conversation, and indeed most of the difficult or uncomfortable situations we have to face in life, is all a matter of phrasing – how to verbally dis-engage from the conversation in a way that you feel comfortable with while getting the point across.

Here are the top exit lines that display tact and grace to give a conversation deer his freedom back:

1. "Oh shoot, I have to say hi to Jessica, I'll catch up with you later!" (act like you urgently need to see Jessica)
2. "Hm, I believe I have to find the bathroom. I'll talk to you later!"
3. "I'm starving, I'm going to go search order some nibbles. I'll let you know if I'm successful!"
4. "I need another drink! I will be back later."
5. "Oh no, what time is it? I have to step outside to make a quick call, sorry!"

Simply interject with any of these at the slightest hint of a silence in the conversation, and you'll be home free! Make sure to show urgency.

As for avoiding being the conversation hunter, that's a more tricky subject, and is going to require you to develop and calibrate your observational skills. Among the things you'll have to learn to develop awareness on are:

1. Are they making eye contact with you or scanning the room behind you?
2. Are they bantering back and ask questions, or are their responses short and unenthusiastic?
3. Are they fidgeting an inordinate amount?
4. Is their body language turned away from you or poised for movement?
5. Are they checking their phone while talking to you?
6. Are you talking more than 80% of the time?
7. Do you frequently hear variations of the exit lines above?

Context is important, but if you answered yes to any of those questions, you just might be a conversation hunter. It's up to you now to realize when your conversation partner isn't as engaged as you are, and either gracefully exit, or attempt to find a superficial or core commonality as I discussed earlier.

If you choose the exit option, you can use the same exit lines that a conversation deer would use.

I more often than not recommend just exiting gracefully because it is the first step to improving the reputation you doubtlessly already have. Not every interaction has to end in a connection, and that's okay.

<u>What your conversation partner will think</u>: (nothing, they will probably be oblivious and looking for their next deer)

Principle 19: Practice Emotional Intelligence.

Emotional intelligence is the ability to accurately identify and manage your emotional state and intent, as well as the emotional state and intent of those around you, in order to achieve better relationships and greater success. Let's unpack that dense definition.

What does it mean to accurately identify and manage your emotional state and intent? When we feel and act out our emotions, we express them first internally to ourselves, then externally to whoever we might be speaking to. However, the internal perception of what our emotions are don't always match up with the external reality of what is actually expressed and projected.

Your emotional *intent*, knowing why you're feeling the way you do, is also prone to mis-identification and mis-attribution. Empathy plays a large role here, because if you are familiar with an emotion, you can better identify it and deal with the consequences.

It could be something as simple as Johnson having a fight with his wife and crankily lashing out at his secretary for forgetting to staple something. What's the true reason for his anger, and how might the secretary know?

We want to believe that we're relatively straightforward and honest, but instinctually we know that there are too many instances in our daily lives that say otherwise. It's just not often that we are 100% transparent with our emotions to ourselves or others. If you can see how mixed up we can be about the emotions that we feel ourselves, you can imagine just how difficult it is to truly sort through the emotional states and intent of other people. Bridging that gap almost becomes an impossible task when viewing it in that context!

And it is a difficult task: friends that have known each other since grade school and confide in each other constantly may not even be able to identify and manage each other's emotional states and intent. However, emotional intelligence is about empathy, reading between the lines, communication, and introspection.

High emotional intelligence is characterized by the following:

1. Understanding your own strengths and weaknesses from an objective perspective.
2. Understanding the exact reason you are upset when you get upset.
3. You are a good listener, and tend to know people's motivations for their actions or words (by dissecting how they emphasizing certain words, use different vocal inflections, and by asking the right questions)
4. You are good at reading people's facial expressions (blinking, tension around brow and mouth, scattered eye contact) and body language

(posture, holding arms or legs, shifting between stances, gestures) to intuit non-verbal messages.

5. You understand and can get along with almost anyone because of your empathy.

6. You also tend to help others because of your empathy, and to an extent, your sympathy.

7. You are emotionally even-keeled and not prone to strong negative emotions because you understand the causes and all perspectives involved.

8. You are a good judge of character and often have a "gut feeling" about people.

Once you can accomplish most of the above, you'll be light-years ahead of that childhood friend and on your way to cultivating your emotional and interpersonal intelligence. The benefits you might notice are invaluable and can be literally life changing.

You'll have deeper, closer relationships with your friends and significant others.

You'll move up more quickly at work because your emotional intelligence will make you a more effective leader and teammate than someone more qualified.

You'll deal with conflict and argue in a more productive, healthier manner because you'll be able to identify the causes, choose your words carefully, and acknowledge all perspectives.

You'll live a less stressful and overall happier life because you'll understand why you feel your negative emotions, and what you can do to rectify them.

You'll begin to be described as charming, great with people, understanding, and easily relatable.

The first step to emotional intelligence is turning a mirror upon yourself and really looking deep.

<u>What your conversation partner will think</u>: It was like she read my mind! She understood things I haven't even told my closest friends.

Principle 20: Conversational Chemistry is Queen, Topic is King.

There's an old saying that goes "The King is the head of a country, but the Queen is the neck and can turn the head any direction she chooses." What's that got to do with small talk, charisma, and forming instant connections?

For all the Principles about choosing and finding conversation topics that flow naturally, cut deeply, and make people expose themselves to you, the conversation topic itself is ultimately secondary.

The *topic* functions very much like the King – it's a figurehead that appears to matter and direct the conversation. But if you can create *conversational chemistry* with your conversation partner, then the conversation topic almost doesn't matter at all. Chemistry is the Queen of the conversation, hands down. Ultimately, you can be talking about diarrhea, as you probably do frequently with your friends, and it won't make a difference. The important part is that you understand and are comfortable with each other. No one can talk about interesting topics 100% of the time, so conversational chemistry is what sustains a connection.

At this point of the book, you should be familiar and comfortable with the simple fact that what matters in a conversation is the connection you're building, and how you end up feeling about the other person – the conversational chemistry. That's the singular goal that the vast majority of my Principles strive to impart. A conversation is a give and take, a dance, and it takes two to really feel true conversational chemistry.

Eye contact, as you've no doubt heard, is extremely important in establishing conversational chemistry.
Next time you go outside, put sunglasses on and try making eye contact with strangers. Now that you can stare with

impunity, you'll notice how many people completely avoid eye contact, and how many simply break it nervously after a quick glance even though they can't see your eyes. It's a powerful feeling, and that confidence and connection translates well into a conversation. Eye contact, like much body language, can make points very succinctly if done correctly. The lack of eye contact doesn't necessarily have to indicate anxiety, it can also show boredom which can be potent.

Body language plays as pivotal a role, but let's focus on my biggest tip without launching into a huge Principle on the typical body language indicators and behaviors. What movie or television show have you seen recently that contains what you would describe as a confident male or female figure? They are now your role model, and it's up to you to compare yourself in a mirror to their strong and welcoming body language.

<u>What your conversation partner will think</u>: Instant friend! He was so funny and had some interesting thoughts on diarrhea. We have to hang out again.

Conclusion

It would be dishonest for me to promise that simply by reading through this book, you'll be a small talk master, ooze charisma, and be able to form instant connections. What I can genuinely say is that you now possess all the tools you need to accomplish your goals and achieve the heights you want, but these are skills, and skills need practice and time.

So when you aren't able to immediately become the life of a party or captivate your next conversation partner, relax and give some of the Principles another read. When the pieces start to come together for you, it is my sincere hope that you are able to reap the benefits of chatter as I have. The results can truly be life-changing, and you'll begin to see how your mastery of the game can easily separate you from others. Good luck!

Sincerely,

Patrick King

Dating and Image Coach
www.didshereply.com

P.S. If you enjoyed this book, please don't be shy and drop me a line, leave a review, or both! I love reading feedback, and reviews are the lifeblood of Kindle books, so they are always welcome and greatly appreciated.

Other books by Patrick King include:

Did She Reply Yet? The Gentleman's Guide to Owning Online Dating (OkCupid & Match Edition)
http://www.amazon.com/gp/product/B00HESY42G

Charm Her Socks Off: Creating Chemistry from Thin Air
http://www.amazon.com/dp/B00IEO688W

The Coffee Meets Bagel Handbook… for Men AND Women
http://www.amazon.com/dp/B00ILATYZS

Cheat Sheet

Chatter Principle 1: Bulletproof Your Nonverbal First Impression.
Start with an impressive handshake, dress and groom to avoid snap judgments, and curate your body language.

Chatter Principle 2: Bulletproof Your Verbal First Impression.
Develop your elevator pitch to the first couple of topics that sprout up in any conversation.

Chatter Principle 3: WWJD? What Would Jay Do?
Channel Jay Leno's singular interest and focus on his guests.

Chatter Principle 4: Your Life is a Series of (Mini) Stories.

Anticipate frequently-asked questions and have mini stories ready in place of one word answers.

Chatter Principle 5: Thorough, Exhaustive, and Specific Details.
Divulge specific and sometimes personal details early and often.

Chatter Principle 6: Icebreak with Superficial Commonalities...
Use icebreakers about superficial commonalities based on gender and mutual shared realities.

Chatter Principle 7: But Core Commonalities Foster True Relationships.
Dig deep to discover core commonalities.

Chatter Principle 8: Know and Play in Your Wheelhouse.
Utilize the Russian doll and atom models to expand your areas of expertise and comfort.

Chatter Principle 9: Reactions are Worth 1,000 Words.

Deduce the emotional reaction that is being sought and deliver it verbally and non-verbally.

Chatter Principle 10: Cold Reads Accelerate Any Conversation.

State a bold assumption that logically flows from something that was said.

Chatter Principle 11: Listening Effectively is like Giving Out Truth Serum.

Paraphrase, re-state words, ask digging questions, and pause for 2 seconds before answering.

Chatter Principle 12: Skew Slightly Inappropriate.

Make an inappropriate but contextual statement to open people up.

Chatter Principle 13: Callback During Conversation Lulls.

Refer to previous statements or jokes during conversation lulls.

Chatter Principle 14: You Are a Current Events Sponge.

Keep up to date on politics/sports/media current events by using your opinionated friends.

Chatter Principle 15: Charisma is a Choice.

Charisma = your presence, genuine interest, and creating pleasure.

Chatter Principle 16: Save Buzzkill Topics for the Internet.

Appeal to the buzzkiller's vanities, then change topics.

Chatter Principle 17: Outrageous Introductions Eliminate Awkwardness.

Introduce people with a funny story about either person or yourself.

Chatter Principle 18: Don't be a Conversation Hunter or Deer.

Make sure you're not cornering people in conversation, and tactfully exit conversations when you want.

Chatter Principle 19: Practice Emotional Intelligence.

Learn the difference between the internal and external emotional expression for yourself and others.

Chatter Principle 20: Conversational Chemistry is Queen, Topic is King.

Focus on creating conversational chemistry as opposed to finding a golden topic.

33677101R00064

Made in the USA
San Bernardino, CA
07 May 2016